Fitness:

The Guide To

Staying Healthy

By

Scott Hayward

Limits of Liability / Disclaimer of Warranty:

The authors of this information and the accompanying materials have used their best efforts in preparing this course. The authors make no representation or warranties with respect to the accuracy, applicability, fitness, or completeness of the contents of this course. They disclaim any warranties (expressed or implied), merchantability, or fitness for any particular purpose. The authors shall in no event be held liable for any loss or other damages, including but not limited to special, incidental, consequential, or other damages.

This manual contains information protected under International Federal Copyright laws and Treaties. Any unauthorized reprint or use of this material is strictly prohibited. We actively search for copyright infringement and you will be prosecuted.

Table Of Contents

Introduction

What does the word fitness mean to you? To each person, its something different. To many it's a word that brings on the cringe of pain, of doing something they simply hate and even something they will avoid at all possible costs. But, that's not necessary for most people.

In fact, fitness can be enjoyable if you know how to make it be just that. Through this e-book, we will teach you several very key elements to keeping yourself fit. Each tip and tool given is something that you can do easily, without much help and with the ability to see benefits.

You won't lose a magical 100 pounds this first three months. You may be able to drop that amount of weight, though, in a year's time. In many ways, fitness can be fun and we'll show you how to make it just that, healthily. Instead of a gimmick diet, another useless fad and any type of crazy health food that costs more than all of the meals from your family, this is a simple, no nonsense approach to overall fitness that simply makes sense.

You'll learn something and you'll be able to implement these tools today to start seeing success. Really, it can be that simple to be healthy. Let's make fitness fun, then.

Chapter 1: Fitness And Where You Stand Right Now

Fitness is a term that is used to help define the ability to stay in the best physical shape. You may ask, then, "What am I staying in shape for?" To each person, this will be something different.

For most, it is a matter of staying healthy as long as possible. You see, your body is designed to work as a machine. When each part of the machine is cared for, the entire machine works the best that it can. When the machine is neglected either in part or in the whole, then the machine won't run well and eventually won't run at all.

If a car, for example, is well maintained for many years, it will last many years longer. If it isn't taken care of, for example you don't change the oil in it, you cut several years off the life of the car. That's costly to you, but when you look at this as your body, you are shaving away days, weeks, and even years off of your life when you don't take care of your machine (your body.)

Fitness is a necessary part of life. Before we get on the soap box, remember that fitness is something that you can get into the habit of doing which makes it easy.

Fitness is not something that you have to struggle with. When you were three you were probably taught to brush your teeth. You learned to put your clothes on. When you were learning how to do them, you likely hated it. But, once you learned how to do it, it became something that you didn't think twice about. Do you worry about brushing your teeth today? No, because it's a habit. That's what we want you to think of when you think of fitness.

It's just something that you do. Granted, the first weeks of learning to be fit and staying healthy will be the hardest. You'll dread it. You'll find excuses about not doing it. You'll claim that getting fit is just too hard. You just can't give up what you love. That's not true.

In fact, if you have the will power to save your life by sacrificing for just a few weeks, you'll see that fitness can be easily mastered by you.

Our first goal is to determine where you stand right now. Don't worry, this is painless, but it may hurt your ego a bit to do it. Nevertheless, it's an important first step.

Where Are You Now?

Take a look at yourself right now. What do you see? If you are unhappy about any part of your body, chances are good that area of your body is bothering you because it's an unhealthy area.

Here are some questions to ask yourself to determine where you stand right now.

- Do you have aches and pains in parts of your body that are not from an injury?

- Do you have clothing that doesn't fit parts of your body well?

- Do you struggle to do physical activities? Do you avoid them because you know you can't do them?

- Are you unhappy with the way that your body looks? Do you avoid looking in the mirror?

- Have you been told by your doctor, your family or others that you need to consider your fitness?

If so, then you need to begin by understanding that change needs to happen. There are several tools that you need to use to determine your health level currently. You can find calculators for many of these available to you free of charge on the web. You need to use them to understand exactly where you stand right now.

- Your Blood Pressure: The pressure in which your heart pumps blood throughout your body. You need this number to be there, but it needs to be in a certain range to be healthy. For adults, this is generally 120 to 139/80 to 89. Ask your doctor where your blood pressure is.

- Body Mass Index: Your BMI is a measure of the percentage of fat on your body. The higher this number is, the more prone to health risks you are.

- Ideal Weight: In comparison to your height and body structure, your ideal weight is the weight that you should be, ideally.

These three things are critical elements for you to take into consideration when considering where you stand right now. But, there's much more for you to consider.

One thing that we want you to do besides getting the above information is to grab a tape measure and get one of the most important measurements out there: your waist.

Your waist is important because it is the indication on your body of your potential health risk. Those that have a larger midsection are most prone to health risks.

This is an important piece of information because of how vital it is to your health. Those that have a large midsection are the most prone to heart problems. The fat that is here will push into your body, causing difficulty for each organ there. Your kidneys, your lungs and even your heart are suppressed. In effect, the fat here is likely to be what kills you, if you are overweight.

What To Start With

To get started with fitness, start by getting through these basic first steps.

1. Meet with your doctor to talk about your overall health. Ask him for measurements of your blood pressure, your heart rate as well as any other important factors he may be interested in you improving. Determine that you are healthy enough physically to begin improving through diet and exercise.

2. Get your weight. Do this at home on a well programmed scale, not at your doctor's office. Do it first thing in the morning after you've gone to the

bathroom but before you have eaten. Do it the same time and same way every time you weigh yourself.

3. Calculate your BMI. You need this to see just how unhealthy you are currently. It's going to come down and that will be quite rewarding!

4. Measure your waist. Stand up straight. Pull up your shirt, suck in your gut and measure at your belly button all the way around using a tape measure. This will be your indication of your weight loss and health improvement.

5. Set your goals. Determine what's important for you to maintain, to improve on, and to work on first. Write them down and post them in several locations in your home.

Now that you have this done, you can begin to improve your health. We'll help you throughout the process!

Its Not Only For Weight Loss

Although many people start looking into fitness because they want to lose weight, fitness is not just about weight loss. By understanding where you stand on these factors above, you can work to improve your overall wellness and increase your lifespan as well as the quality of life that you are currently living.

If you don't think that you need to lose weight, that's great! You are one step closer to being healthy. But, that's not to say that you don't have health problems beyond that level. Many people are still at risk for high blood pressure, high cholesterol as well as other concerns even though they aren't technically overweight. Therefore, you need to take into consideration the fact that overall health is in fact important to improve.

Throughout this book, we'll point you in the direction of improving your overall health. For many that will mean losing weight. For others, that will mean improving other qualities of your life. There's much to learn and improve on for most of us.

What You Will Learn

So, what will you learn through this book?

- Improving your body fitness

- Improving your diet fitness

- Improving your mind fitness

- Improving your lifestyle fitness

Each of these aspects is quite important. While your body must be maintained as much as possible for health, it doesn't do much good if you don't eat the right foods. Losing weight, for example, isn't enough if you aren't eating the right foods even if you are losing weight.

With your mind fitness, we mean making sure you are emotionally and mentally fit. That means insuring that your overall life is healthy in regards to the life that you lead. Emotional stability is critical to overall health.

With lifestyle fitness, the goal is to improve your stress level. It has been shown that those that are under a lot of stress are often the most at risk for health problems due to the stress.

Throughout each of these aspects, we'll teach you how to improve your life through easy, and even fun, ways. Because each plays a role in your overall health, we'll tackle what the healthy standard is, help you to understand where you are and then help you to get to the goals that you have.

Since your body is likely to be your largest factor impacting your life, we will start there. Remember, each aspect is just as important as the next, though.

Chapter 2: Body Fitness And Its Effect On Your Life

Remember how we referred to your body as a machine? Well, the time has come to improve the way that machine is working. This means physically. Your body is a well designed machine, actually. Each part of your body functions well because of the support that other parts play.

Your heart pumps oxygen rich blood to each cell in your body, delivering fuel to is so that it can perform its duty. Your lungs supply your heart with that necessary oxygen. Your brain keeps everything working, even those things that you don't think about doing like your heart beating and your lungs breathing.

Your job is to give your body what it needs to continue to perform correctly. While your diet is something for the next chapter, we need to address your body's ability to do what it needs to through being physically capable.

What some people don't realize is why their body has developed as it has. Well back in the time of the cave man, the body had to do what it needed to so that you could stay alive. It would store food in fat so that when there wasn't enough food available, these fat reserves could be used.

Your muscles are necessary for functioning but they have been built to be used, not to sit ideally. Your body is used to providing your muscles with the fuel that they need to work hard. If you don't work hard, your body can't maintain a healthy muscle mass.

What's Healthy?

As we mentioned early, to know what level of fitness your body is in, you need to take into consideration the vast number of measurements that we've already taken. Your weight, your blood pressure and your body mass index are good indications of your overall health.

Yet, it goes further than this, too. You should understand how well your body is working, too. Do you have any physical limitations? If you physically can't lift things for fear of hurting your back, this could be a potential problem that needs to be considered.

If you have problems with your legs, your neck, your arms or anything else, you should address these specific concerns. The best place to start is to work with your doctor to determine why you aren't physically fit in those areas. That way, you can improve your overall health and then improve upon your situation by knowing how to.

Where Are You?

As we've mentioned, it's important for you to know where you stand health wise. That means taking the measurements that we've listed. You should weekly weigh yourself, the same day at the same time each week. Keep a log of this information so that you can see your progression.

Talking to your doctor is a great place to start when it comes to determining your overall health. You shouldn't skip this step. If you are overweight, chances are good that your heart has been affected by it. You may not physically be able to exercise to a certain level. We won't even include that level of exercise here because your doctor must tell you what's okay and what is too much.

If you aren't having any physical limitations, pains or weight problems, that's a great sign. Now, look at your body in other manners to determine what you can improve on. Even an overall fit person can often improve their body's fitness through improving their body's makeup.

Understanding where you are is difficult for many at first. It's a hard realization. But, it's not the permanent solution, its going to improve, one step at a time.

How Can You Improve

Improving your body means improving your body's ability to move and function. Its not easy thing to do at first, but it will get easier. Our overall plan to improving your body's fitness level is through exercise, coupled with the other fitness elements later throughout this book.

Exercise is something that people hate, but remember your body is built to be used, not to sit in a chair at a desk all day. It is estimated that most people don't get the exercise that they need and that leads to all types of health problems.

Again, even if you aren't overweight, chances are good that you aren't getting enough exercise and fitness into your life anyway. Using your muscles and strengthening them are vital to improving health and fitness.

Aerobic Training

Movement is important for your body. Exercise is the best route to take to gain that health. Aerobic training is the best way to improve your overall exercise tolerance and therefore to improve your muscles.

Aerobic training helps to increase your heart's ability to pump and therefore to get oxygen throughout your body faster. In this type of training, your body will work to improve its function by improving how much work your heart can do.

To find out if you have any limitations, talk to your doctor. If not, then start with a basic program. Here are some tips for you to get in aerobic training.

- Start with basic aerobics and work up as your tolerance increases. Walking is a great place to start.

- Increase your resistance by taking trails that offer hills or speeding up your walk as you improve.

- Move on to more aerobic style exercises. Swimming, bike riding, playing your favorite sport, running, elliptical machines, and other physical activities are perfect for aerobics.

Your goal is to start with 10 minutes of continuous aerobics three times a week. You should try to increase this to 30 minutes three times per week, though, as soon as your body allows for it. The guidelines of your doctor are a must to follow!

Strength Training

Along with aerobic training, you also need to consider adding strength training to your workout. Now, you don't have to be a body builder here. You don't have to have bulging muscles. But, you do want to develop lean muscles that are strong and therefore healthy.

If you need to lose some weight, strength training is a very essential aspect of making sure that happens. With strength training, you will be able to move flabby muscles and fat into lean muscles. Muscle burns through fat faster, allowing you to lose weight faster.

Strength training is essential because it allows you to improve the way that your body works, too. Muscles that are strong are less likely to become injured. They are able to be used easier, with less likelihood of being strained or hurt through your daily exercises, movements or even in accidents.

Here are some tips for exercising through strength training.

- Work with a low amount of weight first. Never increase the weight you are doing unless you are okayed to do so by your doctor.

- Consider working with a physical trainer. This small investment of time and money will allow you to improve your overall muscle mass faster, and more effectively.

- Change up the exercises that you do so that the process is easy and fun. You'll enjoy it and you'll see improvement in the tone of your body quickly.

With strength training, you should add in ten minutes per day three times per week at least. Again, you'll want to increase this number over time to at least 30 minutes per day three times per week. Remember to include ten minutes before and after your workouts for warm up and cool downs!

Your Overall Body Fitness Plan

To improve the physical fitness of your body, you need to give it the physical movement that it needs. This means feeding it the right regimen of movements.

Start by working in exercise through aerobics and strength training into your day. Visit your local recreational center or community center. You can even start doing these things at home, too, which will make the process easier and even more enjoyable.

To make it even better, consider these easy and fun ways to get in the exercise that you need.

- Do it with a pattern. You are 80 percent more likely to be successful if you don't try to do it alone! Recruit someone to work with you!

- After dinner, head out for a walk with your spouse for a few minutes. If you can't leave the kids, take them with you. This is a great way to get in some quality time away from the television.

- If you can't leave the television, use a stationary bike. During your favorite show, ride the bike. You get the exercise you need without missing your television program and time will fly by.

- Do sports and other physical activities that you enjoy. Swimming, playing a game with the kids and even joining a sports team is a great way to get in exercise without it feeling like exercise.

Your overall body fitness means exercise and movement. When you begin to add these into your day, you'll probably find every excuse not to do them. Yet, you will come to enjoy exercising. For many it's a great stress relief and it can be a lot of fun. Make it your goal to actually put together a workout that you enjoy. It will make all of the difference in how effective it is for you.

Chapter 3: Diet Fitness, You Are

What You Eat, Really!

"Diet" is a word that is only second to that of exercise when it comes to hatred by many people. But, here, we aren't talking about a diet to lose weight. We aren't talking about a diet that you will go on to lose weight and then come off of later.

What you need to accomplish through a diet is to train your body to eat healthily. You need a diet that is actually a way of eating, not a temporary thing but a permanent thing.

Although that sounds even worse, dieting is something that is simple to do healthily even if you can't live without certain foods. You can do it even when you are in too much of a rush and don't have time. And, you can do it with lots of favors that you AND your children will enjoy.

Don't think about a diet that's taxing, troublesome, limiting or boring. Think of your diet as being free, open, full of taste and adventure, with all of the comfort that you want and need, too.

What's Healthy?

The foods that you need play a significant role on your health. Foods are the fuel that your body requires to do a good job at the tasks that you ask it. In our machine look at the way that food works, the food that you consume is the fuel that your machine needs.

If you don't give it quality food, it won't perform the right way. Have you ever gone to put gas into your car and gotten to a really bad gas station where the fuel wasn't high quality or even up to standard? It slows your car down. You don't get the gas mileage that you are used to and you may even need to perform more maintenance on your car than you usually need to do.

In the way of your body, healthy food is just as important. If you consume the wrong foods all of the time, your body will not be able to perform as well as if you gave it the highest quality foods.

- Without nutrition, your body can become ill faster and with greater intensity.

- Your body does not heal as quickly from injury.

- Your blood pressure rises, your heart rate increases to unhealthy levels.

- You are more prone to limitations physically as well as mentally.

All sorts of problems arise from not eating a healthy diet of food. But, what is healthy and why is it healthy?

- Vegetables are one of the highest nutrient rich foods out there. They provide antioxidants to a high level that helps to heal your body, improve your physical fitness from the inside to the out, and they are very low in calories meaning you can eat more.

- Fruits are sweet so they can solve the sweet tooth. They also provide you with antioxidants and all types of nutrients that give your body the fuel it needs.

- Whole grains are also an important product of a healthy diet. Unlike "white" foods, whole grains give you so much more health. They don't cause you to gain weight like others. Choosing simple differences from bread to pasta to potatoes allows you to get the tastes that you love but without the added calories, fats, and sugars that can cause you health issues.

- Water intake is also important. Those that do not get enough fluids end up having a body that retains water rather than having less. The body goes into dehydration mode, causing you to keep in all that you can. Consuming enough water means that you'll system is hydrated, you're eating less and that you aren't getting as many calories from other liquids.

- Meats are important parts of the diet, too. You need protein but you shouldn't want to get it from fatty meats. Improving your diet to just lean meats will allow you to cut down on the intake of cholesterol which will ultimately clog your heart minimizing blood flow to the rest of your body.

If you don't do anything else, improving these five areas is all you need to do. The good news is that you don't often need a lot of work to make them happen.

Your doctor may have additional or different recommendations for your health, too. He or she may recommend a diet that is different for your specific health issues. In addition, you may want to find out if there are any possible problems with the foods that you eat to your overall health specifically for your health problems.

Dieting To Lose Weight

Finally, if you need to lose weight, you need to minimize the amount of calories that you are taking in by monitoring how many you are consuming.

The average person should consume about 1800 to 2000 calories per day. If you are dieting and need to lose weight, you need to reduce this amount to at 1500 to 1600 calories per day. Go with the reductions that your doctor recommends here so that you have enough fuel for the day but are not allowing your body to store the extra fuel as fat throughout your body.

Where Are You Now?

When it comes to improving your diet fitness, you need to take into consideration the location that you are right now.

What do you eat for breakfast, lunch and dinner? How many calories are you consuming per day?

To help you to see the clear picture of what's happening to your health in the foods that you eat, take note of how a normal day or week goes for you. Here are some steps to follow to find out how healthy your diet actually is and how healthy it isn't!

1. Spend one or two days recording the foods that you eat in an average day on a piece of paper. All foods and drinks should be noted!

2. Figure out how many calories you are consuming in an average day.

3. Look at your list of foods and see how many of them are high in transaturated fats, sugars and calories in general.

4. How many servings of vegetables and fruits are you getting? How many servings of protein has been lean protein? Did you get in any whole grains? How much soda did you drink (which puts pounds on your waist each time?)

5. How often did you eat without actually being hungry but being instead bored, anxious, stressed or otherwise emotionally impared?

When you look at these facts you may clearly see where the problems lie. Being honest with yourself is important, though. For most people this is as simple as tracking what they eat over the period of a few days to a week.

Seeing just how much in calories as well as in unhealthiness can really cause them to see what reality really is rather than to assume they are doing okay.

I Can't Give It Up!

If you are one of the many that feel that they can't give up the foods that they love no matter what, there are several key things for you to address. Don't worry, they aren't all bad!

First, find out why it is that you can't give them up. For example, are you connected with that big slice of apple pie because it was your favorite growing up, you may have an emotional attachment to the foods. If you love your mashed potatoes loaded with gravy, sour cream and butter just because you love the taste, that's a different story.

Identifying why you have to have a specific food is important so that you can actually see the benefits of eating those foods. If you need apple pie to feel safe, you need to address this emotional problem. If you just love the taste, you can find ways to get much of the same taste without a lot of the calories.

Next, determine if there is a better way for you to get the foods that you like. For example, will sweetened sweet potatoes that are mashed still give you the same texture and creaminess that you are craving?

By making small changes to the recipe you can get all of the flavor and texture that you want without causing yourself to become a victim of high fats and sugars that really do a number on your entire system.

Indeed you may want that slice of apple pie. But, use it in a different way. For example, instead of eating it every few days make it the reward that you get for a week of good eating. Limiting how often you get the treats means that you don't have to give them up but that you don't consume nearly as much of it, and therefore you can improve your health overall.

One limit to this is when the food itself is detrimental to your health condition. If you are a diabetic, you simply should not eat foods that are overall sweet because they can cause your blood sugar level to rise so fast that you can cause serious damage to your brain and your heart through the consumption of just some foods.

You should know what types of foods you can not eat. If you don't know you should talk to your doctor about this. There are certain times in life that foods become prime suspects to leading to health risks. Food isn't worth the risk of your life, is it?

How Can You Improve?

Okay, here is comes. The awful, limiting diet that's going to make your taste buds go permanently bland is up next, right?

NO! You don't have to be limited by what you can eat because most food that is available that is in its natural state is just fine for you! In fact, if you give it a try you may find that you like these foods better than you do the high fat, high cholesterol foods that you currently are eating.

This section of our book is long for a reason. Foods are a main part of why people are unhealthy and therefore it is a mandatory part of improving your health to improve your diet. If you can not commit to making changes here, your diet fitness can threaten your life through disease and even early death.

Yet, much of the damage that is done through eating the wrong foods can be reversed over time by eating a healthy diet. That's exactly what you need to strive for here.

We've already talked about what foods you need to eat for a healthy diet, now you need to consider how you will make changes that you can actually live with.

Here are several key areas to make changes and exactly how you should make them. Don't fret about the foods you love, remember moderation is the key factor in real diet fitness health.

Heart Health

Improving your heart's health is essential. For this, eat lean cuts of meat. Paying attention to the amount of saturated fats in the food you eat is also key to improving your health and well being.

In addition, there are various foods that can help you to improve your hearts health. For example, replacing the vegetable oil in your diet with olive oil, in moderation can improve your health. Garlic is a great antioxidant for your heart too. Reducing the amount of sodium that you take in is also a key factor in improving health. Instead of using a lot of salt, try other flavor additions to your dishes.

1. Consume more fish. You should try to consume at least 2 to 3 servings of fish per week. Or take a supplement of fish oil.

2. Eat unrefined whole grains as they add fiber to your diet which reduced your cholesterol and keeps you feeling full.

Improving Health Risks

Another very powerful tool that you have when it comes to diet fitness is that of improving your health through the foods that you eat. Your weapon is that of antioxidants!

Antioxidants are powerful nutrients that are in fruits and vegetables. A good way to know if they are in the foods that you are eating is to look at the color of the food. The darker, richer and brighter the color is, the more antioxidants are in it.

Antioxidants can help to transform your health. They can help to repair damage to cells throughout your body and thereby make you look and feel younger. They can help to unclog your heart's arteries from cholesterol. And, they help to remove toxins from your body which means a reduction in risks of cancer.

Using antioxidants for your overall health is a key factor in improving your health! While you can get many of them through supplements, you should instead consider getting them from whole foods as they are richer as well as tastier that way!

Eat Whole Foods

One of the best things that you can do for your health is to eat whole foods rather than foods that are pre-made. Yes, you are in a hurry and who has time to chop up vegetables? Well, there are reasons why an investment in a bit more time here can literally save your life.

Many foods that are pre-made contain high amounts of preservatives, or products that are placed in foods to keep them fresh and looking good. Some of these preservatives can clog up your heart, can lead to increased health risks for cancer and they put the pounds on.

The trick you should follow, then, is to visit your grocery store and walk around the outside aisles only as much as possible. No boxed dinners, no frozen entrees. The produce section is your friend filled with riches. Meats, milks, eggs and other fresh products usually line the walls of the building. Avoid the aisles and you'll improve your health overall.

Overall Diet Fitness Plan

Does this sound like a lot of work? Don't worry; we'll make it simpler for you. Here are the tips that you need to get your diet fitness plan off the ground and allowing you to improve your health considerably!

1. Eat more fruits and vegetables. Visit your favorite recipe sites on the web and look for vegetable recipes that aren't rich with sauces, butter or creams. Add one new recipe to your diet each week.

2. Start looking for leaner cuts of meat. Remember, meats that are high in saturated fat are clogging your heart. One good switch is with ground meats. Don't reach for beef, but replace at least part of it with ground turkey or pork. You won't notice the taste difference. Eat more fish, chicken and pork over beef.

3. Reduce portion sizes. No food in one sitting should be a larger quantity than the size of your palm. To help you to not feel hungry, eat a bit slower.

4. Visit the website of the American Heart Association to get heart healthy recipes. Try to look for ways to improve your current recipes through replacing butters, salts, unhealthy foods with foods that are better for you. Look at your grains. Replace white rice and pasta with whole grain. Replace white bread with whole grain bread.

5. Remove soda from your diet. This single movement alone will improve your health considerably. It adds

weight to your body and it causes all types of health risks later in life.

6. Look at labels. Learn to read labels so that they tell you what's in the foods you eat. Reduce the amount of fat, cholesterol, and sugars in the foods that you eat.

If you need to lose weight, then you need to consider a calorie reduction. Dropping just a small amount of weight means that you need to eat less and do more physically. There is no fad diet that is more comprehensively safer and effective than just that: eat less and get more exercise every day.

Eating healthy isn't an option if you wish to increase your lifespan and increase your health. While you may love food, learning to make healthier recipes shouldn't be something you put on the back burner because you are too busy, don't like those foods (you probably don't know what they taste like anyway!) or you think its too much work.

Food is a requirement to living and a healthy diet is an essential part of living a long life. Don't make sacrifices here for speed, convenience or habit. Remember; while making changes at first is a challenge, you will get into the habit and will eventually love the differences you have made, guaranteed!

Chapter 4: Mind Fitness, A Healthy Emotional Life

As you can assume, your mind is a powerful tool and it helps you through each step of your day. It controls the way that you perform each action, the way that you see life and it controls all of those little things like breathing and your heart pumping that you don't think about.

Yet, there are many ways that your mind's fitness may not be the right level that it should be. In fact, for many people living in today's hectic lifestyle, it's anything but easy to make it through the day without dealing with some type of stress or pressure.

The mind's health is quite an important aspect and, believe it or not, plays a significant role in the quality of life and the longevity that you have in your life. When you are emotionally or mentally unfit, your body's health is directly related.

There are many different ways that this can happen, including the simple fact that you may have to battle illnesses more often and with greater intensity.

Although you may be wondering just how you can control your minds fitness, the good news is that this can be one of the easier steps to take in total health and wellness if you allow it to be.

Let's get started by learning what exactly is healthy and what may not be the best choice for your overall health and well being.

What's Healthy?

For your mind to be in a healthy state, several key things must play a role. First, you need to be fully capable of thinking clearly; performing mental tasks and you need to be able to conquer problems effectively. In addition, you need to tame those other things that happen throughout your life that limit you or otherwise affect the quality of your mind and lifestyle.

A Healthy Brain

With the onset of Alzheimer's happening to more and more people, the importance of having a healthy brain is very evident. Whether or not you can stop this disease or other debilitating diseases from happening to you is yet to be seen, there is evidence that says that you can actually push off the onset by some time if you do the right things.

For this particular battle, you need to exercise your mind. Keeping your mind active, challenged and attentive is essential to your well being and this fight.

Emotional Health

Another aspect that you probably don't want to talk about is that of emotional well being. While life affects each one of us, the way that you handle the problems that happen to fall into your lap are critical in maintaining a healthy life. For example, should something emotionally troubling happen to you, such as a death or deception, you need to be able to effectively deal with it and then to move on.

Emotional health is an important battle that everyone must strive to improve. There are many various ways that you can improve your emotional state by learning how to react to critical situations. Indeed, the right social activity is one way to improve your emotional health.

Stress Management

Yet another factor that plays a significant role in the well being of your mind is that of stress. Not only does it pull you down through causing large amounts of emotional trauma, but it also causes all types of physical problems for those struggling with it. It can lead to various health issues physically, too.

While you can't take away everything in your life that causes stress, learning to effectively manage stress is important. It can help you to tackle even challenging tasks with more ease and with success. Sometimes it may be important to remove the stressors from your life, but that's not a common occurrence.

Spiritual Well Being

Spiritual well being is yet another consideration that you need to take. While there isn't always a need to be religious or spiritual, it can often play a role in the way that you see your life as well as in your emotional state of mind. For those that do believe in a Higher Power, the need for spiritual well being is even more evident because it places a significant role in your self esteem and your outlook on your own life.

Spiritual well being is a critical factor in maintaining your health, too. Those that are spiritually fit, feel good about themselves which allows them to be more likely to improve and maintain a healthy lifestyle.

This is a personal decision, of course, but aren't all of these aspects of fitness personal decisions that you need to commit to? Spiritual health is something to think about.

Where Are You Now?

When it comes to determining how mentally fit you are, you may think that you have nothing to worry about. After all, you do all that you need to do and there's nothing limiting you. But, have you actually reached the highest level that you can?

Usually people struggle with this aspect because of the vast number of misbelieves about mental and emotional well being. Believe it or not, most people go through stages of depression, mental turmoil and even times when they are so stressed that they can not function properly. During these times, you can consider them, and you, mentally unstable and unfit.

Yes, it hurts to hear but just like your body goes through illness, your mind can be struggling at the same time, although you may not realize it.

To determine where you stand in mind fitness, ask yourself these questions. Be honest, now, there's nothing for you to be embarrassed about but a lot to be gained when you can improving your mind's fitness.

1. Do you have physical pain that is not the result of an injury? This could be stress related!

2. Do you struggle with remembering things from one moment to the next? Do you find yourself struggling to remember why you walked into a room?

3. Do you struggle to make the goals that you set for yourself?

4. Do you feel anxiety, stress and angry often? What does it feel like and how intense does it get?

5. Do you hate the life that you are leading, are you unhappy with your lifestyle or do you have regrets about your life?

All of these things play a role in how mentally fit you are. While you may not want to do this, you should schedule a meeting with a psychologist just to talk through some of the feelings that you have. For the most part, working through these issues can be the best way for you to overcome your problems and to find overall benefit in your life.

If you have trouble sleep, or are eating whenever you feel like it, then you should be considering the vast number of mind fitness needs you may have.

Improving the fitness of your mind not only improves your daily life but increases your longevity, too!

Emotional Eating

We touched on this subject just a few minutes ago in our dieting chapter but it's important for you to address now, too. Emotional eating is eating when things go bad, when you are stressed or when you are in the mood for a certain feeling that you can't get from the world around you.

For many millions of people, this is one of the prime reasons that they are overweight or unhealthy in their diets. While food never used to be so readily available, today its easy to have a pantry full of food and a refrigerator that's stocked to the brim. It's easy to go to the food to get the satisfaction that you need.

Yet this is a dangerous situation. Those that use food to fight their emotional instability are most likely to fall deeper into a path of self destruction. For example, consider this scenario that happens over the span of time.

You begin by getting stressed at work. You find yourself reaching for a candy bar to get the extra rush that you need to get through the tasks at hand. You then find yourself dealing with pressure from the boss; you didn't do the job right. You decide you need a big, fatty lunch. Soon, the pounds are creeping onto your hips. There's no time to exercise and to meet deadlines you increase the amount of bad foods you are eating. Soon, you are not fitting well into your clothing. You become upset at yourself, your self esteem drops.

As your self esteem drops, you find yourself in even more problems. Now, you hate your job so much that the only thing that makes it feel better is eating something bad for you. In fact, you almost purposely make the situation worse by eating bad. You aren't any good. You are a failure. You can't make the right decisions. Just look at you….these are all things that people end up saying to themselves when they are emotionally depleted.

Emotional eating is one of the hardest cycles to break, yet if left intact, it's also one of the worst things you can do for both your physical and your mental health state.

In just a bit we'll talk about some of the ways that you can have good mind fitness, which includes emotional eating. The first step in fighting the way that food makes you feel, though, is to recognize that there is a connection between the way that you feel and the way that you eat. Realizing this makes a large difference in improving both your physical fitness and your mind's fitness.

How Can You Improve?

How can you improve your mind's fitness? There are many great ways to make this happen. Remember when we said this fitness plan was going to be fun? Here there are many great ways to improve your emotional and mental fitness through fun methods.

Each aspect is unique in itself and in the way that it will help to improve both your physical fitness and your quality of life. Incorporate as many of these things into your life as you can, and you'll see differences in the way that you feel and the way that you see the world.

Your Self Esteem

We'll tackle one of the hardest things to improve right from the beginning: your self esteem. A health self esteem is one that's confident but not overly macho. You should be able to feel confident in the decisions that you make and in the way that your life is moving. Confidence is built on many things including the fact that you have to realize that you do have weaknesses and you do have limits to your abilities. Accept those, work on improving them if you can and then do the best job that you can overall.

In addition, learn how to accept compliments and to take criticism. Getting down on yourself because someone doesn't like the job you did isn't okay.

Although challenging, you need to be able to say, "Hey, I did a good job!" You also need to recognize when it wasn't your best work and realize that it's okay not to be perfect 100 percent of the time. Learn to take criticism positively. If your boss says that the job wasn't good enough, ask what you could have improved on for next time. Then, you set yourself up for success rather than a pint of ice cream!

One way to improve the way that you look and feel about yourself is to take care of your outward appearance. Those that dress well, take care of the way that they look and those that do things for themselves are the most confident people out there. Just putting on a beautiful outfit can make you feel good about yourself.

Build A Social Network

A social network is a very important to your well being, both physically and mentally. Those that have people around them to support them do well in many more aspects of their lives. Let's face, its fun to have people around too! But, how can you build a social network of people that you can rely on?

Make time for those that you already have. Don't assume that they will always be there when you need them, even when you don't pay attention to them otherwise. You should always strive for a lifestyle that's positive with those in your family and your friends. That means taking on the challenges that come up between people, working through them and then letting them go.

Relationships take time and work. If you are married, that relationship alone will be one that you have to work on. Realizing that you aren't always right and making sacrifices for those that need you to can be an important and difficult risk you have to take.

Commit to going out and having fun, whatever way is fun to you, at least one time per week. Getting away or even just finding time to play a board game is essential. This allows your mind to repair damage and it allows you to improve your network of friends.

Don't take friends for granted because they won't be there when you need them the most. In part of that comes the fact that if you want to have family and friends you need to be a friend, too. Giving others support helps them to accomplish their life's needs and it gives you a sense of gratification. You'll feel good about life and your social network.

Managing Stress

Its not easy job, but you have to do it! Stress is one of the largest problems in health today. Stress affects your ability to function properly. It hinders you throughout your life by causing unhealthy living situations, physical risks and puts your entire well being at risk for emotional breakdown.

To help remedy stress, there are many things that you can do. For starters, find an outlet. You need to find something that you love to do. A hobby, a physical activity, or some other thing that really brings you happiness is necessary to have. By doing that activity even after a long and stressful day it can offer you improvement in your health and well being, by relieving stress.

If the situations that you are in provide you with high levels of stress, it is important for you to find solutions to those problems. You need an effective manor for relieving stress and if you can't do so by solving the problem or by letting go of the stress you need to remove yourself from such situations. Stress that is ongoing without any real stopping is a large health risk!

Brain Power!

To improve mental fitness, use your brain power! You don't have to do any type of exercise with your brain physically of course, but mentally you do!

For starters, always keep yourself learning. Learning new things keeps the mind active and that means health. Someone that is learning new things that interests them is likely to continue to having a mental state that's positive and motivated.

You should also use challenges to help power you through your day and your life. Giving yourself the ability to overcome challenges from puzzles to problems in life (yours or others) can help to keep your brain working. Asking questions, getting the answers and working at it helps to improve the brain's function, allowing you to fend off Alzheimer's and other conditions like it.

Your Overall Mental Fitness Plan

So, now you have it! You know what to do to make your lifestyle improved through these changes. Here's a quick look at the changes that you can make today that will increase your mind's power later and throughout your life.

1. Improve your stress levels and see physical, mental and emotional benefits right away.

2. Improve your social network to reduce stress and to improve your quality of life. It also helps to make it through difficult times when you have someone by your side.

3. Improve your brain's fitness by challenging it through new adventures, continuous learning and through challenges of all types.

4. Do things that are enjoyable to you. If you can't think of anything, learn something new. New adventures coupled with doing them with those that you love make life better and help to improve your mental fitness.

5. Keep your self esteem positive. Working on this is hard, but feeling good about yourself is a must for overall health.

By doing these things it will significantly improve the fitness that your mind has physically and emotionally. The good news is that you can change the outcome of your day by just making the right decisions on the way to look at challenges during the day. Make changes like these today and see results today.

Chapter 5: Lifestyle Fitness, You Are What You Do, Too

Your lifestyle is the way that you live your life. Although each of these other elements that we've already talked about is very important parts of your lifestyle, they are not everything.

Each decision you make throughout the course of the day plays a role in your fitness. Unlike the other chapters, this one will be structured a bit different. Each of these lifestyle considerations is important and each offers a unique spin on the quality of life you will lead. Improve them, and physical fitness increases.

Smoking, Drinking And Drugs

Each of those three things, smoking, drinking and drugs, is a problem for your health and your ability to make it through the life you have. You probably already know the risks of what these things can do to your life, but you may not realize the extent at which it takes to improve them.

For example, smoking will eat away at your lungs and will cause cancer. There are no ifs about it. It will cause cancer eventually in your lungs.

But, smoking is something that you can stop, even if it is one of the hardest things you will have to do. To improve your fitness, find a method to stop smoking and do it. You will find that your health increases, your energy increases, your stress levels DO go down and you can feel better about the life you are living.

When you quit early enough, your body can repair the damage that you have done to your lungs. This can only happen if you stop soon enough, though.

Drinking and drugs are just as bad. Each time that you consume too much alcohol that makes you drunk or you take illegal drugs, you destroy your body slowly and methodically. You kill brain cells, you put your life at risk and you destroy the organs in your body. Some damage can be fixed through healing over time, others can't.

To improve your lifestyle and to extend your life, you need to remove these problems from it. Smoking and drugs are simply a no no. Drinking alcohol isn't nearly as bad for you when you drink it in moderation and only when you are drinking low concentrations of alcohol such as in wine rather than in hard liquor or beer.

Sleep

Do you sleep? No, we mean actually lying down and sleeping for 7 to 9 hours per night? Do you wake up rested? If not, then you aren't getting the right amount of sleep for health. Your lifestyle fitness requires that you get quality sleep each night.

Why is sleep so important? There are actually several reasons. For one, sleep is the body's time to relax and to recoup what it's done all day. You need this time for your mind to. It's the way that your mind works through problems. It's the time that your body heals from the exertions of the day.

It's a time to restart, refresh and give yourself the best chance at improving tomorrow.

Those that don't get enough sleep are not capable of performing at their best physical or mental level. They aren't able to improve the level at which they can function and they make bad mistakes. Stress hurts more, physical ailments hinder you more when you don't get enough sleep.

If you are having problems with sleeping, there are many ways that you can overcome them.

- Reducing stress levels during the day is helpful as is working out the stresses that you can't get rid of.

- Try to go to sleep at the same time everyday and give yourself as much time as necessary to feel rested.

- Don't do stimulating things before bed such as watching television or working on a project.

- Don't eat before bed, at least two hours beforehand.

If you are facing problems with insomnia or are struggling to get to sleep, talk to your doctor about it. There may be an underlying medical condition that could be causing it.

While it used to be that there were only sleeping medications that were addicting, today there are many that are not like that which can offer you a night's rest. Don't use these unless your doctor has Okayed them for you, though!

Supplements

Giving your body the nutrients that it needs to make it through the day is essential to your well being. But, even if you think that you can do this through the foods that you eat, you are probably still missing out.

Today's foods often do not contain enough of the nutrients that your body needs to be in your best physical shape. While a diet that's full of nutrient rich food should not be replaced, it sometimes needs additional supplementation to take it to the best level it can be at.

But, what do you take? First off, find a good quality multi vitamin and take that as directed. Multi vitamins are a good starting point because they provide a decent dose of supplements that just about everyone needs. Multi vitamins give you what your food doesn't and they are affordable solutions to your needs.

In addition to this, find out what type of supplements you can take for your individual needs and problems.

For example, if you have a need to lose weight, look for supplements that can offer weight loss benefits.

If you have heart problems, problems with gaining weight or other conditions, you can probably find a supplement or several that can address those problems for you.

How do you know how much to take? That's a trickier question. There are two routes to take. First off, realize that doctors don't always use supplementation in their practices and they may not be educated in prescribing this type of help to you.

First, start by finding a health food store or a vitamin supplier. Quality is very important if you want to see benefits from supplementation. Therefore, make sure that you have a reliable source. These individuals can also help provide you with the information you need regarding improving your conditions.

Another source for information is the web. Finding a reputable website that offers help for supplementation will help you to increase your overall well being through tackling individualized problems. Again, quality is essential to success here. Don't assume that any information that you find is reliable. Get another opinion!

Supplements can help to improve your body's function because you are giving your body exactly what it needs to do the work right. It's like always giving your car premium gas and oil to do its job even better!

Financial Concerns

Getting your finances in order doesn't seem like it would be a lifestyle change for fitness benefits, but it really can be. Just think of the role that money plays in your everyday life. You worry about money and end up facing financial hardships that move into your work life, your home life, your marriage, and even your physical health.

Financial fitness isn't something that we'll stress for too long here, but it is something to make part of your overall guide to living a long, healthy lifestyle.

As you know, stress causes a wide range of health concerns for your body. Money is one of the largest causes of stress in people every single day.

Therefore, when you want to improve your well being and health you need to take into account the fitness of your overall financial life. In the perfect world you would have plenty of money to do what you want to do. But, that's not always possible.

So, to help you, we've put together some things that can offer you success when managing your financial outlook even when you are struggling to make ends meet.

- Live within your means. While it's nice to have what everyone else has, its not going to make your life better to have them. For example, if your neighbors just purchased a new car, you may feel like you need to have one too. But, will having a new car really improve your life? Then it may not be worth the financial risk and cost to own one.

- Don't use credit. Credit today is used for everything from buying a house or car to buying lunch at McDonald's. While you may need to use credit for the larger, more expensive purchases, keep as many of your other purchases credit free. This may be hard, but if you stop using credit today and start using cash, you may find yourself with more cash to spend then credit!

- Make a budget with your entire family. It goes without saying that you can't spend what you have if you don't know what you have. Each month make a goal of tackling one extra bill to pay it down as much as possible. Give yourself some money to use as you want for entertainment each month too, so that you don't feel deprived. You are more likely to stick with your budget this way. Include each family member in the making and keeping of the budget!

- Don't eat out. This isn't good for your waistline anyway! You can save thousands of dollars each year by eating at home! You'll cut the pounds off, eat better quality foods and better recipes!

Getting your finances in check may mean talking with various people including your lenders and financial planners. But, if you didn't have to pay all of those credit cards each month, how much money would you have in cash to spend? Get to that point and you'll have immeasurable success throughout all areas of your life, too.

Meditation And Yoga

There are many ways to improve the quality of your life, but one that you may not have thought of is that of meditation. Some don't believe it can offer them benefits but there is one thing that meditation and yoga can definitely provide to you: the ability to relax.

Yoga is a great tool for both exercise and relaxation. Both meditation and yoga have been shown to provide improvements for those that are in need of stress relief. And, when you learn how to do them effectively, it takes minutes a day to wash away your stresses.

So, how does this fit into your lifestyle fitness plan? It's simple. You need to spend ten minutes each day, usually before breakfast, quietly meditating or doing yoga. Ten minutes per day is all that it takes to see significant improvement in your overall well being.

When you take into account all the things that you are doing in the morning you may not think you have time. But, again, invest the time for a couple of weeks and you are sure to see the improvements quickly and they will not be such a demanding time taker.

You can learn how to do either meditation or yoga (or both if you like) easily. Some people are familiar with it enough that they can learn how to do is through at home study. It's often a better solution, though to learn with others through a professional.

Get together with a friend and take a class at your local recreation center or your community college. You'll find that once you learn the technique you can do the process on your own, easily.

Rewards

How does reward play a role in the life that you live? How do rewards actually help you to improve your lifestyle fitness? It may seem strange to include them here, but the basis is very simple: rewards help to keep you going and they make life worth living. It's that simple.

In each of the various things that we've talked about in this book, there are countless different sacrifices that you'll have to make. Some small, some large, but each one needs to be met in order to give you an overall well being and healthy lifestyle.

It's hard to give all of that up, that's for sure. But, one thing you need to keep in mind is that the struggle isn't for nothing. You will find rewards at the end of the struggle when you have improved your life and removed the toxins and troubles from it.

Yet, from point A to point B is a long road. To help you through it, dedicate some time to rewarding yourself along the way.

For example, if you are working on your physical fitness, give yourself the reward of a day at the spa, a night out on the town or even buy yourself something when you obtain your goal or one of the goals along the way.

While you are dieting, you can reward yourself too, in the same way. Its important not to overdo it with rewards of food that are unhealthy, though. But, you can definitely give yourself a bit of your favorite dessert if you've eaten well all week!

When you obtain your goals or the stepping stones to your goals, give yourself a bit of a reward. It makes life a bit sweeter and makes the hard work that you've been doing much more successful and worthwhile. Those that reward themselves stick with the program longer and eventually do better in the long run, too!

Conclusion

The process of improving your life is one that takes time and dedication. Improving your body, your diet, your mind and your lifestyle is a complex process. And, it will mean stumbling along the way.

The best route for you to take is the one that's most important to you first. Perhaps you need to concentrate on one aspect first such as your diet and then later incorporate your body fitness, your mind fitness and your lifestyle fitness goals.

You may be able to pick one of each of those category's goals and work on each one. You may be better off looking for rewards by taking it one step at a time.

Your first goal is to make your own goals. What do you want to improve in your health and well being first? Write down your goals and keep them with you and place it throughout the house. Recruit a family member or friend to work with you, too. Improve your life one step, one healthy change at a time and you'll reach your goals.

The reward is health, a happy life, one that's full of fitness of your body and your mind and one that's rewarding to you and to the rest of your family. It a process worth working for, and soon you will see that isn't anything worse than brushing your teeth and putting your clothes on each day!

To your fitness!